Vitamin D Diet Benefits

Sunshine, Best Foods, & Disease Prevention

By Peter Kornfeld
Copyright © 2012

© 2012 by Peter Kornfeld

ISBN-13:
978-1481851206

ISBN-10:
1481851209

First Printing, 2012

Printed in the United States of America

Income Disclaimer

This book contains business strategies, marketing methods and other business advice that, regardless of my own results and experience, may not produce the same results (or any results) for you. I make absolutely no guarantee, expressed or implied, that by following the advice below you will make any money or improve current profits, as there are several factors and variables that come into play regarding any given business.

Primarily, results will depend on the nature of the product or business model, the conditions of the marketplace, the experience of the individual, and situations and elements that are beyond your control.

As with any business endeavor, you assume all risk related to investment and money based on your own discretion and at your own potential expense.

Liability Disclaimer

By reading this book, you assume all risks associated with using the advice given below, with a full understanding that you, solely, are responsible for anything that may occur as a result of putting this information into action in any way, and regardless of your interpretation of the advice.

You further agree that our company cannot be held responsible in any way for the success or failure of your business as a result of the information presented in this book. It is your responsibility to conduct your own due diligence regarding the safe and successful operation of your business if you intend to apply any of our information in any way to your business operations.

Terms of Use

You are given a non-transferable, "personal use" license to this book. You cannot distribute it or share it with other individuals.

Also, there are no resale rights or private label rights granted when purchasing this book. In other words, it's for your own personal use only.

Vitamin D Diet Benefits

Sunshine, Best Foods, & Disease Prevention

Table of Contents

Introduction

Did you know that in Canada, approximately 97% of the populace is deprived of adequate amounts of Vitamin D in the winter? It is really astounding! And what's even more peculiar is that even in warmer climates like Southern California, people don't get enough Vitamin D from the sun to protect against disease.

And further still, if you reside about the 38 degree north latitude, running straight through Denver, San Francisco, St. Louis and Baltimore, you get almost zilch sunlight in the winter months.

It goes without saying that Vitamin D is something that your body needs to stay healthy. In fact both your body and mind require regular amounts on a daily basis. This can be in the form of natural sunlight, which is preferable, diet or supplement form.

Up first we are going to uncover the deep, dark secrets of Vitamin D (just kidding).

Benefits of Vitamin D

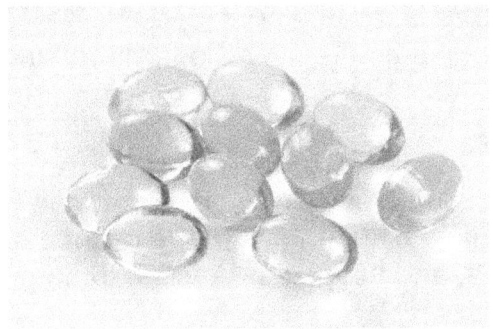

I'm going to start off by explaining in brief what Vitamin D is, so that you understand things from the ground up.

Vitamin D is a steroid, specifically a group of soluble pro-hormones, which encourage the absorption and metabolism of calcium and phosphorous. Fair enough?

Now it's safe to say if you expose yourself enough to sunlight without sunscreen, under normal circumstances you'll get all the Vitamin D required.

And were you aware there are five different forms of Vitamin D? They are D1, D2, D3, D4, and D5; the most important of which is Vitamin D2 (ergocalciferol) and Vitamin D3 (cholecalciferol). Don't worry about memorizing those names because I'm not going to quiz you, at least not yet! The idea is to be familiar with them; that's all.

But before we move on, we're going to have a look at

these five types a little closer. This will help you to see
the important role Vitamin D plays in your body and life

as we know it.

VITAMIN D1

Is referred to as a molecular compound. And as mentioned above, it attributes to ergocalciferol and lumisterol.

VITAMIN D2

This vitamin is derived from ergo sterol. And we're going
to expand a little bit here. It is made by invertebrates, and
various plants and fungus, in reaction to natural sunlight.

We, as humans do not make Vitamin D2 and the role it
plays with invertebrates isn't well known. But one thing
we do know is that ergo sterol is an excelled absorber of
UV light, which causes harm to DNA, protein and RNA.
This is one reason many experts agree that sunscreen
helps protect us from the damage caused by the sun.

VITAMIN D3

This vitamin is actually synthesized in your skin when 7-
dehydocholesterol meets with UV light. The UV index
must be greater than three in order for this to happen;
which just means there is a certain threshold of sunlight
required for the production of Vitamin D3.

To give you a better idea, UV levels of three or more are
all the time in the tropics, throughout spring and summer
and some of the time in the fall. Although in the arctic cir-
cles you will hardly ever hit this target.

Experts agree that we need at least 15 minutes of exposure to the sun at bare minimum two times a week, without sunscreen. If you get too much the vitamin supply just diminishes.

We will talk a little more about this particular vitamin in a later chapter, so you're going to have to hold your horses for now.

VITAMIN D4

Otherwise referred to as 22-dihydroergocalciferol.

VITAMIN D5

It is made from 7-dehydrositosterol, otherwise known as sitocalciferol. Got all that?
 Ok, now we are going to get into a little of the meat and potatoes.

Some of the Other Benefits of Vitamin D Are:

* Helping take care of our bones. Here, Vitamin D helps encourage the metabolism and absorption of phosphorous and calcium.

* Helping to regulate our immune system functions. What it does is act like a natural antibiotic supplement which helps fight off colds and other minor infections; making sense of the fact that most colds and flu are evident in the winter time, when there is less natural exposure to sunlight on a daily basis.

* Deterring specific diseases from developing. For example, Vitamin D may lower your chances of facing the challenges of multiple sclerosis. Interesting how this disease prominence is much lower the closer you get to the tropics, where there is more sunlight.

* Decreasing the incident of colds and flu. Scientists agree that by strengthening your immune system with adequate bouts of Vitamin D, you are less likely to deal with colds and sickness in general.

* Helping to keep your weight in check. Believe it or not, this vitamin plays a primary role in helping to regulate your system and maintain a healthy weight.

* Encouraging your cognitive capacity to increase. Studies have shown that getting adequate amounts of Vitamin D will help your brain and thinking process stay clear and strong as you age.

* Assisting in lessening the symptoms of asthma and other breathing disorders. This makes sense because with a strong immune system, asthma is less likely to be triggered.

* Reducing the risk for women of developing rheumatoid arthritis. Experts agree there is a protective mechanism that is triggered with adequate intake of Vitamin D.

* Lowering the risk of various cancers. Again, studies indicate that Vitamin D has beneficial effects in bettering the outcome of people with cancer, and lowering the number of people developing it.

* Reducing the damage caused by low level radiation to the body. This of course is extremely helpful for people receiving radiation therapy when fighting disease.

Some more advantages of Vitamin D are:

* Children and young babies that go into the sun on a regular basis are less likely to get stuck with a cold.

* When the flu season peaks during the winter months, there is substantially less sunlight available to expose yourself to.

* During the warm summer months, the flu virtually disappears.

* Using UVB sunlamps, which of course make Vitamin D in the skin, reduces that bouts of colds and flu in children.

* In large doses, Vitamin D will help boost the overall health of children, especially those prone to sickness and infection.

As you can see, adequate amount of Vitamin D are extremely beneficial to your wellbeing as a whole.

My Thoughts . . .

The more in tune you are with your body the better it will treat you. That's just the way the cookie crumbles. Vitamin D in adequate amounts is essential in helping you maintain your health. Understanding it is a critical element in the 'big picture.'

My thoughts are why wouldn't you make certain you get lots of Vitamin D each day? You are important and making Vitamin D a priority just makes sense!

Now we will have a look at sources.

Sunshine is the Best Source!

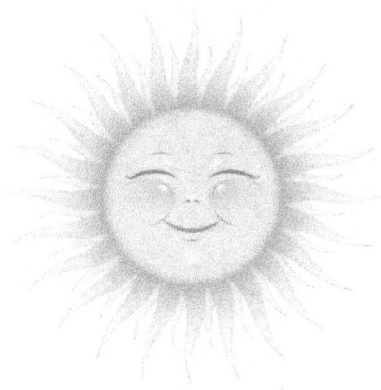

Hands down the best source of Vitamin D is to get your bare butt out into the sunshine! Of course everything in moderation is always wise.

The sun is your most effective means of getting Vitamin D. The sun triggers production of it in the skin in response to UVB rays. Guidelines suggest about 15 to 20 minutes of fun in the sun minus the protection each day.

The UV needs to be adequate, which is above three. This will manufacture approximately 10,000 international units in a light-skinned person. What isn't clear though is exactly how much sunlight is required for disease prevention. The jury is still out on that one.
And I'm sure you've heard the UV rating on the radio or seen it on the television before. So it's pretty easy to

know what it is each day.

Of course there is variation with everyone. Dark skinned people are able to naturally manufacture less Vitamin D than their lighter skin neighbors.

Now this is by no means a ticket to become a sun goddess, because there is too much of a good thing when it comes to the sun. Of course there are the risks of sunburn or overexposure to sunlight. And the damage is caused if you go overboard.

And natural is better with most everything in life, wouldn't you agree?

Getting your Vitamin D from the sun is convenient and it doesn't cost you anything, which is most definitely a bonus. You just need to make a point of getting adequate amounts, not under, or over doing it.

Because you will damage your health if you get too little or too much sunshine for prolonged periods of time.

Never forget that a little bit of sunshine really is the best medicine for your health, happiness and positive state of mind!

My Thoughts . . .

Who doesn't love sunshine? And you really can't go wrong with natural can you? Sunshine makes you feel good by elevating your mood naturally.

I'm sure you've noticed that on a day when the sun doesn't appear, people in general tend to be a tad grumpier. It's funny how that is.

18

And my belief is this is linked to deprivation of you much needed daily jolt of sunshine!

Now you may be wondering what sort of foods is high in Vitamin D!

Best Foods of Choice for Vitamin D

I'm sure you've noticed a whole slew of foods that are fortified with Vitamin D in the grocery store. Things like orange juice and milk come to mind. Setting synthetic and supplement sources aside for now, here are some great foods oozing with natural Vitamin D

BUTTON AND SHIITAKE MUSHROOMS

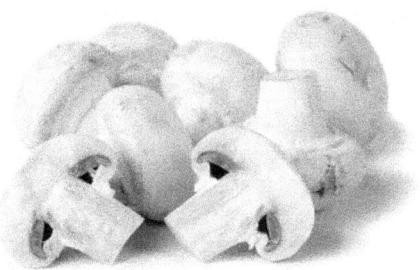

It may surprise you that dried mushrooms have excellent levels of Vitamin D. It is perhaps in part because mushrooms thrive from sunlight. And it is critical the dried mushrooms you choose have been dried with natural sunlight and not artificial; simply because artificial sunlight will diminish their Vitamin D content.

SOCKEYE SALMON

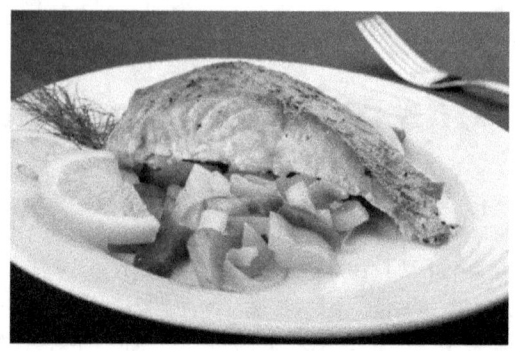

Did you know that just one 3.5 ounce serving of salmon will give you nearly all the Vitamin D you need for the day? Make note this salmon needs to be wild because the zooplankton these fish eat helps to boost the Vitamin D levels.

MACKEREL FISH

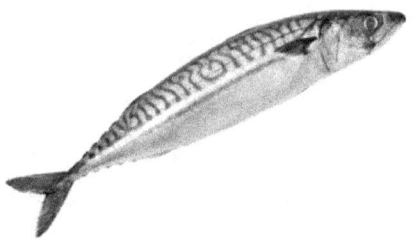

The oils and Vitamin D from this type of fish is fantastic for your health. And suffice to say, just one serving of mackerel will give you up to 90% of the recommended daily intake you require of Vitamin D.

TUNA

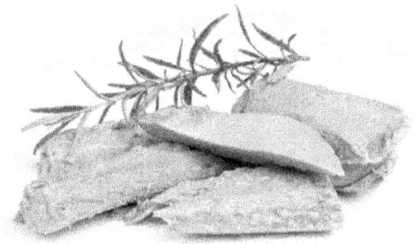

 Natural wild tuna is the best. And with just one 3 ounce serving you can get about 50% of your Vitamin D for the day. Not too shabby I must say! And the bonus here is the oily fats will help with memory and your cognitive capacity.

EGGS

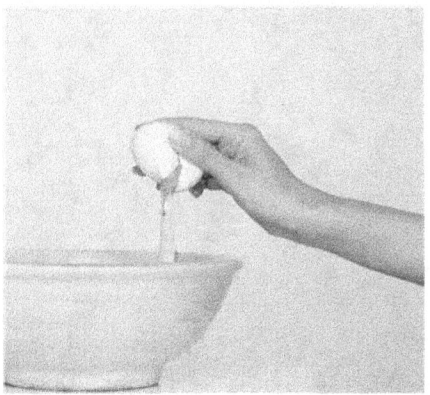

Interestingly eggs are also a good source of Vitamin D. Eating one egg will give you about 10% of your daily Vitamin D needs. You do the math as to how many eggs you need to make the grade!

Again it's best to eat eggs from free-range chickens as much as you can.

SARDINES

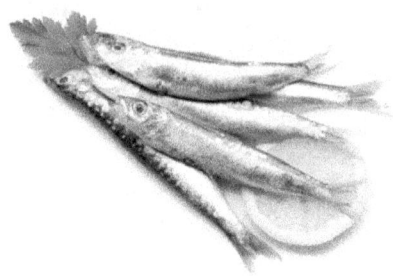

With sardines most love or hate them. If you love them, you are in luck with the Vitamin D stuff, because a can contains about 70% of your daily requirement. Wow!

CATFISH

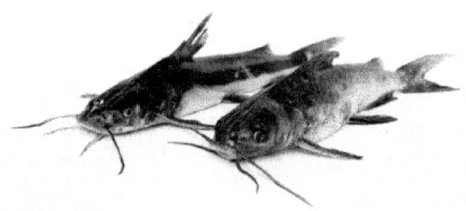

These critters are likely a great choice because they enjoy feasting on plankton. This helps make them another prime source of Vitamin D.

COD LIVER OIL

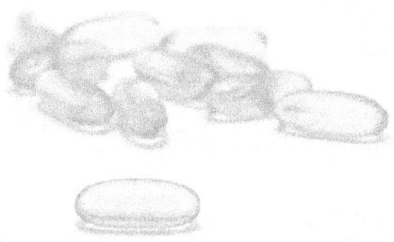

Yuck! Sorry. I had to say that. I remember my grand-mother telling me horrific stories about having to take spoonfuls of cod liver oil growing up!

And if you can stomach it, cod liver oil is incredibly rich in Vitamin D. It also contains numerous important fatty ac-ids. And if you can keep it down, it will help sharpen your thinking, improve your nervous system, and contribute to strong and resilient bones.

One tablespoon is enough to do it for you my friend!

As mentioned before there are some fortified foods readi-ly available to you. But before we get into examples we are going to look at what exactly fortified foods are.

Turning back the clocks almost a century, salt was the first food fortified. This was manufactured in 1924, where salt was fortified with iodine to prevent goiter. Of course since then many foods have been fortified with various vitamins and minerals, in order to lower the risks for seri-ous health conditions.

The reason for Vitamin D fortification is because of a need for more Vitamin D intake for most of the popula-tion.

Some of the common foods fortified with Vitamin D are:
* Milk
* Orange Juice
* Yogurt
* Infant Formula
* Margarine
* Butter
* Breakfast Cereals
* Cheese
* Soy Beverage

It's important not to assume these foods will give you all the Vitamin D you require. Better is the mindset these foods will top up what you need.

My Thoughts . . .

There are a multitude of food choices that are going to help you get the Vitamin D you need each day. All of them are yummy too, except maybe cod liver oil, but you don't have to have that!

The idea here is to experiment with different food choices, so that you are always varying the quality and quantity in which you get this requirement. That will help ensure you get what you need because your body is always changing and it really can be tough to keep up with them sometimes.
Your body absorbs some foods better than others and this makes diversity advantageous.

Variety is the key in everything, including your vitamins!

That said we are now going to look into measurements.

How Much Vitamin D Do You Really Need?

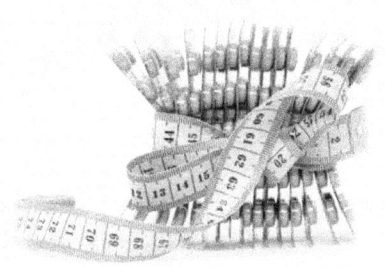

Experts agree the amount of Vitamin D you need daily is dependent on your age.

Infants - Under six months - 400 IU/day - But stay below 1000 IU/day

Infants - Seven to twelve months - 400 IU/day - Stay below 1500 IU/day

Children - One to three years - 600 IU/day - Stay below 2500 IU/day

Children - Four to eight years - 600 IU/day - Stay below 3000 IU/day

Children and Adults - Nine to seventy years - 600 IU/day - below 4000 IU/day

Adults over seventy-one years - 800 IU/day - below 4000 IU/day

Pregnant and breastfeeding women - 600 IU/day - stay below 4000 IU/day

So this gives you a good idea of the amount of Vitamin D you need to stay healthy. And keep in mind none of this is written in stone. In fact as I write experts are leaning towards increasing the recommended daily amounts for everyone significantly.
What isn't clear though is the amount you need to prevent serious disease. Research is ongoing to determine an accurate measurement, being careful not to get too much into your system.

My Thoughts . . .

Now there are always going to be discrepancies in what amount of Vitamin D experts recommend each day. That one is pretty much unavoidable because each one of us if different.

You metabolize Vitamin D differently than I do for instance. And that's important in the big picture. But I think you get the just of the guidelines. Listen to your body, keep ready to get informed, and you can't go wrong!

Up next is a look into one of the D vitamins specifically

Vitamin D3: Up Close and Personal

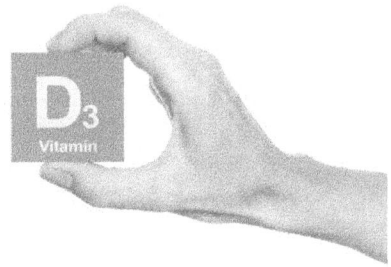

Nutritional experts believe that Vitamin D3 is the simplest nutritional tool we have to help better our overall health and wellness. This specialty vitamin is derived from 7-dehydrocholesterol; but gains hormone mimicking actions when Vitamin D3 is transformed into Calcitriol, complements of your liver and kidneys.

When in hormone form, Calcitriol directs calcium, phosphorus, and bone metabolism, along with neuromuscular function. That being said, Vitamin D3 is the only vitamin that your body can manage from natural sunlight.

Our problem as a society in general is that we live a lot more indoors than our ancestors. And extensively use sunscreen because of the dangers of overexposure to the sun. Because of this we are blocking Vitamin D and creating huge deficiencies in bone strength and immune issues.

Scientists have known for hundreds of years that Vitamin D3 specifically is critical in healthy bones. Further studies show the importance of this vitamin in reducing bone breaks.

Along with this, having a deficiency in Vitamin D3 also shows a link to serious disease including depression, diabetes, chronic back pain, cancer, poor immunity, pregnancy pre-eclampsia, and macular degeneration.

There is no question that Vitamin D3 is imperative in overall great health. But the flip side is people are worried. They don't want to get too much sun because the detrimental effects of overexposure can be deadly over time. This confuses people and often encourages individuals to short themselves on the Vitamin D3 they need to stay healthy, in order to avoid sun damage. Sad but true.

Another factor to consider is where you live. People that reside in climates with minimal sunlight likely need more Vitamin D3 than is recommended.

In fact, as mentioned previous, researchers are calling for higher doses to be stamped in as daily minimums. Inevitably this takes time and more research is needed to back up this finding.

Here are some of the other Vitamin D3 names you may come face-2-face with:

* Cholecalciferol
* Carlson D
* D 1000 IU
* D2000
* D3-5

* D3-50
* D400
* Delta D3
* Enfamil D-Vi-Sol
* Liquid Vitamin D-3
* Maximum D3
* Replesta
* Thera-D 2000
* Thera-D 4000
* Thera-D Rapid Repletion
* Vitamin D3

My Thoughts . . .

As you can see, there is a whole lot of importance behind Vitamin D. And what's critical here is that you take your lifestyle into consideration and make adjustments in your life to get your stores up!

Why?

Well because it's essential in your overall good health. It will help keep your bones limber and strong, and boost your immune system to battle and win against the free radicals we force our body to deal with each day.

Are you with me?

OK, next up we are going to dig a little deeper into what happens if you ignore everything I've been telling you.

Vitamin D Deficiency

So what's a Vitamin D deficiency?

Well if you want to get technical about it, it's when your blood levels of Vitamin D3 are chronically low for a long period of time.

If this was the case, you would be tested specifically for 25-hydroxyvitamin D3.

Furthermore, you'd be surprised just how common Vitamin D deficiency is. And it makes sense that people who live in colder regions, more northern areas, or have darker skin, may be in a higher risk group just because.

Keeping in mind that nobody is immune to this. If you aren't getting adequate sunshine or getting enough Vitamin D from food sources, then you could very well be in need of more Vitamin D.

But that's just the surface my friend because not having enough of this vitamin in your system for a prolong period of time greatly increases your chances of battling over three dozen illnesses head on; including cancer, rickets, Alzheimer's and Osteoporosis.

Think prevention my friend, and by getting the Vitamin D you require on a daily basis, you could very well be protecting your body against these life threatening illnesses.

What's also critical is that lacking this vitamin for long periods of time might be exaggerating the symptoms of issues you are already dealing with. Here you could consider such issues as depression, anxiety and HIV.

There are diseases in which having adequate amounts of Vitamin D are critical. If you don't, then you are only escalating your discomforts and the progressions of the disease. Common illnesses like Multiple Sclerosis, Fibromyalgia and HIV fall under this realm of thinking.

So what are the symptoms?

Glad you asked because the more you are aware, the earlier you can catch this and deal with it, which may be as simple as stepping out in the sunshine a little more.

If you are experiencing bone pain or muscle weakness, this could be your body telling you to up the Vitamin D. It is important to keep in mind the symptoms are often barely noticeable, so you need to have your 'spidey' senses on.

A few more symptoms are:

* Tiredness
* Muscle cramps
* Joint pain
* Chronic pain
* Elevated blood pressure
* Headaches
* Unexplained weight gain
* Bladder issues
* Issues with bowels

It is so very important to be aware because having low levels of Vitamin D in your blood can be intertwined with:

* Asthma

* Various cancers
* Cognitive illness
* Increased complications of cardiovascular disease

What's more, is that experts agree Vitamin D plays an intricate role in preventing numerous conditions from surfacing. These are inclusive of MS, Diabetes and high blood pressure.

Of course the cause of this deficiency is of vast importance.

Here are a few common reasons for lack of Vitamin D

* ***Not getting enough Vitamin D over time*** - This often happens if you are strict with your diet. Maybe you are a vegan and a lot of the food sources for this vitamin are animal based.

* ***Sun worry*** - If you take sun precautions to the extreme and don't allow yourself any time in the sun, you could very well have a deficiency. As you know, your skin makes Vitamin D when in the presence of the sun. No sun - no Vitamin D production.

* ***Darker skin*** - If you are lucky enough to have darker skin, you may not realize you need a little more sun exposure to absorb adequate amounts of Vitamin D. Studies dictate that older adults with darker skin more often have a deficiency here than lighter skinned people.

* ***Overweight*** - If you are obese, you are more likely to have a Vitamin D deficiency. Vitamin D diffuses into your blood from your fat cells. And if you are fat, chances are pretty good you've got a low level of Vitamin D.

* ***Issues with your digestive tract*** - If you have health

issues with your digestive system, your body may not be able to process the Vitamin D you require as well. These illnesses include cystic fibrosis, and Cohn's disease.

* **Kidney issues** - As you get older, it is harder for your kidney's to transform this vitamin into a useable form. This of course increases the risk of developing a deficiency.

Now if you suspect a deficiency, a simple blood test can be performed to find out. If you find a level of 20 - 50 nanograms/milliliter, you're considered healthy here. And if you have a level less than 12 ng/ml, you definitely need more Vitamin D.

My Thoughts . . .

More often than not, a Vitamin D deficiency is a result of people just not being 'in tune' with their body and just not understanding the importance of Vitamin D in their life.

Everyone metabolizes Vitamin D differently depending on weight, age, absorption, health status and how much time you spend in the sun.

And just not being aware of that you need more Vitamin D is good news, because this means with a little more sunlight and some adjustments in the food you eat, you can get rid of your deficiency for good.

Believe it!

Now we are going to look into different Vitamin D supplements.

Common Vitamin D Supplements

Simplified, up to 600 IU per day is required for the average person. And a little more for seniors is a good idea. Up to 800 IU per day is a sound suggestion.

That said, the verdict still hasn't been reached, as to whether or not this is enough to maintain good health and prevent disease.

Reason being, recent findings indicate Vitamin D influence a broader array of physiological processes. Not just bone health and calcium absorption. In fact, current research findings strongly suggest we need more! Up to 5, 000 IU per day in some instances!

That can be tough to get with sunshine and in your diet. And here's where supplementation comes to the rescue.

Vitamin D supplements come in two forms:

* Cod liver oil based - Which is fat soluble Vitamin D. Found in gel caps or liquid drops.

* Lanolin based - This is a dry powder, water-soluble form. Available in tablets or capsules, whichever suits you best.

Experts support the fact that both fat and water soluble Vitamin D are processed; absorbed, and utilized equally by your body.

Vitamin D supplementation should not be your sole form

of attaining adequate amounts of Vitamin D. It should be used in addition to eating foods chalk full of the vitamin and your daily safe-sun intake. Remembering a few minutes of unprotected sun is good for you, but don't overdo it.

Now you may be wondering how you should take your supplement. Chances are you've taken a medication or vitamin before that either had to eat with food or on an empty stomach, if it was going to be absorbed properly.

Luckily both types of Vitamin D can be taken any time, with or without food. If you are worried about absorption, you can always take it with a meal. This will help it stay in your body a little longer, although the directions on the label aren't going to suggest taking it with food.
Another important factor to understand is that your body is built to store Vitamin D. So some people opt to take it a few times a week in higher doses. In other words both daily and weekly usage is equally effective.

There are some precautions you should also be aware of.

You need to speak with your health care provider if you are dealing with:

* Hyperparathyroidism
* Eating disorders
* Granulomatous TB
* Cancer

It's just better to be safe than sorry.

And when it comes to mixing medications and Vitamin D, there are a few things you should know.

First, is that Vitamin D is not known to cause any adverse reactions with Vitamin D.

However, there are medications that will cause issues with the absorption of this vitamin. A few of them are:

* *Various Steroids* - These can impair the absorption of Vitamin D, resulting in the bones weakening and developing osteoporosis.

* *LoCholest and Xenical* - Are both recognized for pushing Vitamin D through your system before it's absorbed properly.

* *Dilantin* - Can increase the metabolism of your Vitamin D to inactive compounds.

My Thoughts . . .

Vitamin D supplementation is an excellent method of making sure you give your body enough each day. It's readily available at your supermarket, or local pharmacy to start.
And what's important is that you understand taking a Vitamin D supplement in most cases, is a great thing. And for some people, without the supplementary option they wouldn't get the Vitamin D their system requires to function optimally.
Ensuring your stores are topped up at all times is going to increase the probability that you are en route to a healthy and happy life!
Let's have a closer look at various diseases and Vitamin D:

Diseases Treated and Prevented With Vitamin D

Believe it or not, lack of Vitamin D plays a role in a whole range of minor and major illnesses and disease. This includes various cancers, osteoporosis, elevated blood pressure, cardiovascular disease, obesity, rickets and diabetes.

Along with various immune diseases, MS, arthritis, gout and infertility, Parkinson's and depression, psoriasis, Alzheimer's, Fibromyalgia and periodontal disease also make the list.

Ever wondered what the most common disease due to lack of Vitamin D is?
Well in children, it's rickets. And a symptom of this is the bowing of the legs, I'm sure you've seen that before. And for adults it's osteomalacia, which is basically a weakened skeletal system.

Rickets

Technically speaking rickets is a fairly common disorder that is a result of inadequate amounts of Vitamin D, phosphate, and/or calcium. And what happens is your bones literally get soft and weak, causes all sorts of problems for you.

Add to this an increased risk of this happening if you live in a colder climate, stay indoors, are lactose intolerant, don't consume milk products, or are a vegetarian. It must also be said that acquiring rickets in a developed nation is really quite rare.

Osteomalacia

As mentioned previously, this illness is basically a softening of the bones that occurs over time. This can happen
because of the lack of Vitamin D, or in some instances
your body may have issues breaking Vitamin D down and
using it efficiently.

Osteomalacia may be developed because:

* Lack of Vitamin D in the diet
* Not enough exposure to sunshine
* Inability for your intestines to absorb the vitamin proper-
ly
* Cancer
* Metabolic issues
* Kidney disease
* Liver disease
* Lack of phosphate in the diet
* Issues with seizure medication

To diagnose this condition you would need blood tests to
measure the Vitamin D in your blood first. Then a bone
biopsy would indicate if you have any bone softening.
And a bone density procedure would show if you've lost
any bone and how severe the bone softening is.

Here are a few facts about Vitamin D and Cancer

* Vitamin D is needed for strengthening, growing and re-
pairing your bones; along with helping in the absorption
of calcium and bettering your immune system. This is all
necessary in deterring cancer from forming.

* Studies indicate that larger doses of Vitamin D from
supplementation, sunshine and/or food, are attributed

with lower risks of colorectal cancer.

* Experts suggest Vitamin D is connected with lower risks of breast, pancreatic and prostate cancer, but more research is needed to solidify the evidence.

* The NCI or National Cancer Institute is still sitting on the fence with regards to the links between Vitamin D and cancer. This means more evidence is required to validate the positive relationship between Vitamin D and cancer.

There have also been isolated studies performed in specific geographical areas. They have found that people in areas prone to more sunshine, seem to have a decreased risk of developing certain types of cancers. This makes sense because you and I both know sunshine is required for natural Vitamin D production.

Other specific studies have discovered that cancer cells in laboratory tests that were given large doses of Vitamin D, grew slower than cells that didn't receive any.

In a little more detail, we are going to have a look at the evidence of Vitamin D and the reduction of specific cancers.

Colorectal Cancer

What the studies found here was that it isn't just the Vitamin D intake that's important here. Yes these experiments indicate increased Vitamin D in your diet seems to reduce the likelihood of colorectal cancer specifically. But the amounts required for this benefit vary case to case and are very difficult to establish.

Here's a little more explanation.

The majority of colorectal cancers arises from pre-existing colorectal adenomas. And anything that reduces this risk of adenoma development, like Vitamin D, has a good chance of helping to lower the risk of colorectal cancer.

Breast Cancer

One issue with a large majority of these studies is that the women participating were taking low doses of Vitamin D, hence the results were more neutral than anything else.

Researchers do believe that if the amounts of Vitamin D were higher for prolong periods of time, the evidence would heighten statistically.

Prostate Cancer

With this one, experts seem to have a mixed bag of evidence to work with. Some studies have shown that an increased dose of sunlight shows a decreased risk of prostate cancer. However some experts have found that too much Vitamin D intake can actually increase your the risk of prostate cancer.
So it's important to gather information from various sources and make the best choice for you.

Esophageal Cancer

This type of cancer is more common than one might think. In the United States alone, about 17, 000 people are diagnosed, and 15,000 die each year.

Studies have shown that statistically, Vitamin D is a viable treatment option to consider. By getting regular direct sunlight you will decrease your risk of developing this type of cancer.

And with the treatment aspect, what happens is that Vitamin D can actually block and prevent the spread of esophageal cancer. All great news when it comes to treating and preventing this type of cancer.

Pancreatic Cancer
Again there are mixed results here in the relationship between Vitamin D and pancreatic cancer. One study that followed over 100, 000 participants for over 16 years, found those with a higher Vitamin D intake had a lower risk of developing this cancer.

However, another smaller study with a little over 500 subjects followed over 12 years, showed an inverse result. In other words this study indicated in increased risk of battling pancreatic cancer with higher Vitamin D absorption.

A little bit controversial, and confusing if you ask me!

But there is still so much research to be done. It looks as if Vitamin D helps promote differential cell structure, lowers the growth rate of cancer cells and instigates apoptosis.

What Vitamin D does is bind to the VDR, which is located in the nucleus of the cell, and is a gene transcription regulator. Vitamin D might very well trigger the increased production of a detoxifying enzyme. This would support the protective role Vitamin D has with reference to cancer of the colon.

Detailed Diseases Positively Influenced By Vitamin D

It's true that Vitamin D has been shown to prevent a whole realm of diseases, but the fact is, it's only been qualified in treating a few. We're going to have a look at a few of these in a little more detail.

The problem here is that it is difficult to reverse the damage any disease has already done. But it is most definitely possible to help stop and slow the damage process in most scenarios. That's why there are only a few illnesses that can truly be treated with Vitamin D specifically.

Sickle Cell Pain - This is a blood disorder, where red blood cells are abnormal. This causes a shorter life span. These abnormal cells tend to block blood flow; this causes pain, infection and damage to your organs.

Studies have shown that large doses of Vitamin D have been shown to reduce and treat the pain caused by this disease.

Multiple Sclerosis - MS is an inflammatory illness where the myelin sheaths around the axons of your central nervous system are harmed. What was found with large doses of Vitamin D, was that over prolonged periods of time, the disease seems to be slowing. Leading researchers do believe that large doses of Vitamin D are helpful in treating the symptoms and progression of this disease. More research studies are necessary to validate this finding.

Various Cancers - What researchers have discovered are large doses of Vitamin D interfere with some cancer cell progression, slowing the growth of the disease. Although the results are promising, a lot more research is needed to unquestionably validate the treatment of Vitamin D for cancers.

Alzheimer's - What's interesting here is that many of the factors linked to dementia and other cognitive disease, are attributed to low Vitamin D stores. To keep things simple, there is a plaque in the brain called amyloidal beta that's linked directly to the progression of Alzheimer's.

Studies indicate Vitamin D may in fact help clear the brain of this, assisting in treating this disease. Again, a whole lot more research is required here but the findings are promising for everybody.

Tuberculosis - TB is a recognized global health problem and studies have found that Vitamin D is extremely beneficial in the treatment of it. What the vitamin does is help suppress intracellular growth; it also induces the amount of cathelicidin involved, which is a defense in TB patients.

Diabetes - There's lots of evidence pointing to 'yes,' Vitamin D can be used in the treatment of diabetes. Diabetes is considered a multi-factorial disease in which both a genetic and environmental factor is present. Experts have found in numerous studies that Vitamin D will help increase the effectiveness of insulin and decrease the severity of inflammation.

These are both encouraging in using Vitamin D for the treatment of diabetes.

It's also important to note that it is pretty much impossible to get too much Vitamin D in your system. This is important to note because there are a wide range of vitamins that can cause serious issue if too much is consumed over a long period of time.

My Thoughts . . .

Although there is a whole lot more research required, the findings thus far in how Vitamin D can be used positively in the treatment of disease, is very promising. It is important to keep in mind that no two people are alike.

Neither is their health condition or the way their body works.

This means that what works for one may or may not work for another. Vitamin D is one of those universal things that everyone needs, day in and out. This means we all start on a level playing field.

After this, all the pieces of information you gather have to be articulated together, and it's you that is responsible for making the decisions as to what works with you. This in-cludes using Vitamin D specifically to treat and more importantly prevent disease.

Working with your healthcare specialist, doing a little re-search on your own, reading e-books, and discussing with friends, family and colleagues, is going to give you the wealth of information you need to make certain you use Vitamin D positively in your system.

Bettering your current situation and helping you to gain control of your health.

 Ok, we are going to take a step in the direction of human physiology and the role Vitamin D plays at the various different stages in life! Are you ready?

Lifecycle and Vitamin D

Infants

It makes sense to start youngest to oldest. Wouldn't you agree? As you well know, this vitamin helps the body use phosphorus and calcium, and helps build healthy bones.

What many people know is that breastfed infants especially need Vitamin D supplementation. Reason being is because although this vitamin is stored in the mother's body for some time, after about 4-6 months of breastfeeding, the supply is depleted. This means the infant is no longer receiving adequate amounts through breastfeeding alone.

With an infant, because they are so small, the amounts need to be fairly precise. Too little can lead to rickets and too much can also cause issues. And because newborns don't get the sunshine when very young, this makes it more important to ensure they get the Vitamin D to help them grow up strong and healthy.

The recommendation is that all infants under the age of a year receive 400 IU of Vitamin D daily. The liquid is generally brownish and color and fairly sweet, so the infant will love sucking it up. A dropper is the best method of administering it, ensuring they get it.

Adolescent

Interesting, there seems to be a deficiency of Vitamin D in female adolescents, especially during the winter months. If an adolescent doesn't get or absorb the proper amounts, there could be consequences including:

* bone mass accrual alterations
* weakened muscles
* cardiovascular issues
* obesity and insulin issues
* neurological disorders

400 IU per day is recommended if the adolescent isn't getting enough. And in some instances as much as 1000 IU per day may be required. Geographical location, skin color, diet, and numerous other issues should be considered to make sure the proper amount is being received and utilized. A blood test can confirm this if need be.

Adults
We are lucky that Vitamin D is available to us naturally, through sunshine. And that our body can store it. But we need to be careful to assume we are getting, and more importantly absorbing what our body needs.

For example, let's say you need a cup of milk and you drink five. This doesn't help you one bit if your body isn't able to absorb the nutrients from the milk, like if you're lactose intolerant. Does this make sense? In this scenario you could drink ten gallons and still not get the vitamins you need.

Well the same thing applies with Vitamin D. So it's important for you to understand what this vitamin does for you, and what to look for if you aren't getting adequate amounts into your system.

Most people get adequate doses of Vitamin D from a combination of sunlight, food and supplementation if required. And there needs to be two hydroxylation's in the body in order for the process to be complete.

What happens first is the liver will transform Vitamin D into calcidol. The next transformation takes place in the kidney, where it becomes physiologically active and ready to go!

This process is needed for bone growth and a healthy skeletal system to start. Vitamin D also helps in controlling cell growth, contributing positively to immune function and reducing inflammation. Cell health is directly associated with healthy Vitamin D stores. And as adults, it is important we maintain adequate amounts in our body, so our body can perform optimally.

A simple blood test can tell you whether or not your body is absorbing adequate amounts of Vitamin D. If not, you can look into taking a supplement in bulk amounts, a few times a week, or in lower doses daily.

Having at least 50 ng/ml in your blood is considered a healthy range.

You can do this because your body can store Vitamin D.

Seniors

Did you know that up to 70% of people over the age of 70 aren't getting enough Vitamin D? That's a shocker for me. And there are a variety of reasons for this including:

* Inability to make Vitamin D because of skin changes
* Unable to get into the sun - nursing homes
* Less likely to eat foods with Vitamin D
* Decline in cognitive area - forget to take it
* Intestines may not absorb as well anymore

The easiest way to check levels is a blood test. And if supplementation is required, usually 800 IU per day is adequate.

And something quite common with the elderly is serious fractures. But by simply maintaining bone health, much of this can be avoided. Of course this means getting all the vitamins and minerals needed is a must, including adequate amounts of Vitamin D.

As with all health issues, prevention is the key and it starts with awareness. Knowing what you need and making sure you get it.

If the elderly doesn't get adequate amounts of this Vitamin their bones will weaken, muscle will be lost, memories will fade quicker, and their immune system will be compromised. None of which is good.

My Thoughts . . .

Vitamin D is just one tiny piece necessary in the circle of life. And it's important you take the time to make sure you have the proper quantities in your system. This isn't something you want to find out 20 or 30 years from now. We need every advantage we can get in the game of life and by making certain you are absorbing the Vitamin D you need, you'll be one step ahead of many others on the quest to great health!

Your overall good health is a multi-factorial component, requiring balance and continuous fine tuning. Are you getting the Vitamin D you need?

How Does Vitamin D Work?

To start, we refer to it as Vitamin D because over time we've created a need to have it nutritionally. Interestingly, in its natural form it's a hormone manufactured and utilized by your kidney.

When exposed to sunlight it is transformed into pre vitamin D. This pre vitamin is transformed into 1, 25 dihydroxyvitamin D by your kidneys, so it's ready to use. Your kidney's then ensure calcium and Vitamin D are used efficiently.

And when you are absorbing the sunshine, previtamin D and Vitamin D break down so you don't get your levels to a toxic high.

When you get enough sunlight to make this vitamin, your body soaks it up through DBP, or Vitamin D-binding protein.
Looking into how your body absorbs Vitamin D through food is a tad bit more complex. But we'll give it a shot!

Your body soaks up dietary Vitamin D like it would cholesterol. What happens is your bile breaks down the lipids, which deliver the vitamin to your fatty tissue. Your liver steps in next to clear it and have it set to be metabolized.

It then ensures you have enough in your system by reading the amount in your blood, what amount is utilized by your intestine, followed by the amount reabsorbed back into your kidney when urine is being made.

Now that wasn't that bad was it?

My Thoughts . . .
Most people would rather not venture too far into the technical aspect of things. That in itself is a whole separate language!
What is important is that you have an ideal of what your body does with Vitamin D, because this will help you better recognize if you are getting the amount you need each day to function.
Information is knowledge and the more you know the better off you will be in the long term.

FAQ's

There are always questions people have that just don't ever seem to get answered. Here are some of those questions that may be hiding somewhere deep in your thoughts.

Do Formula Fed Infants Need Vitamin D Supplementation?

Infant formula is enriched with about 400 IU of Vitamin D, so supplementation isn't needed.

What Risks Are There With Inadequate Vitamin D Intake For Babies?

- Bone growth issues
- Immunity problems
- Development of other diseases

How Much Sunshine Is Required?

Balance is key here my friends. If you get too much you could develop skin cancer and look older than you are. But too little could mean you are getting your needed daily dose of Vitamin D.

In general, if you aren't lacking the vitamin, about 15 minutes in the sun without protection each day is adequate. Just use your noggin!

What Are Good Vitamin D Food Sources?

- Wild fish including salmon, halibut, tuna, and sardines.

- Fortified foods like milk, eggs, yogurt, premium orange juice and various cereals.

- Eggs, specifically the yolk.

- Mushrooms that have been dried, Shiitake.

Just to give you an idea, you need about four servings of fish, or twenty cups of fortified orange juice to get your daily intake through your diet. The sun is looking pretty good don't you think?

Can I Use A Tanning Bed To Safely Get My Vitamin D?

This is not recommended because studies are conflicting as to the safeness of these tanning beds. The light isn't natural and it just shouldn't be used for your Vitamin D consumption.

What Are The Main Symptoms When Not Getting Enough Vitamin D?

- Tiredness, muscle weakness and pain
- Cramping, joint pain and weight gain
- Head pain, increased blood pressure and poor sleep
- Bowel issues, lack of concentration and bladder issues

What Are the Major Diseases Associated with a Deficiency?

There is a huge range of diseases that are both directly and indirectly related to Vitamin D. Some of which are:

- Various cancers, Osteoporosis and Cardiovascular disease
- Increased blood pressure, obesity and Diabetes
- Arthritis, MS and Bursitis
- Fertility issues, PMS and Parkinson's
- Anxiety issues, depression and Alzheimer's
- Psoriasis, Fibromyalgia and periodontal disease

Can I Get Too Much Vitamin D?

Well you can rest easy because you can't get too much of it through sunshine. However, if you went crazy with Vitamin D supplementation for a long duration, you could reach toxic levels. But the chances of this happening unintentionally are like finding a needle in a haystack!

How Much Vitamin D Should I Have In My System?

Normal ranges are between 50-80 ng/ml. Of course this is dependent on your ability to absorb it and your overall health condition.

My Thoughts . . .
The only silly question is the one not asked! I'm sure you've heard that one before right?
Here's where I get the chance to remind you of how important it is to ask questions if you have them. Do a little research, ask your healthcare provider, and do what you need to in order to get your questions answered.

Doing this is going to help you build up your confidence and knowledge base. Giving you the 'knowhow' to make sure you get and are processing all the Vitamin D your body requires.

So let's have a look at the role of Vitamin D in Pregnancy

Vitamin D in Pregnancy

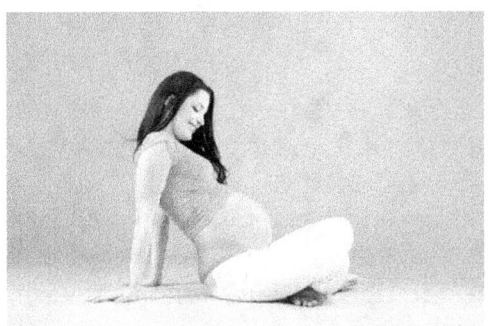

Before we get discussing the effect of Vitamin D in pregnancy, here are a few lifestyle issues that will play a predominant role in how it effects you:

* Skin color - darker skin doesn't absorb as much
* Sunscreen – blocks Vitamin D from being manufactured
* Clothing - hats and outer clothing
* Location - northern climates don't have as much
* Pollution - smog decreases Vitamin D

Ok, understanding this is not an exact science. Especially when pregnant it's important you get all the nutrients your body needs, including Vitamin D.

As it is, Vitamin D deficiency is hugely widespread, a real health issue for many. And unfortunately the deficiencies in pregnant woman may be exaggerated because of the extra demands of the growing fetus.

It's also important to understand that babies who get their nutrients from breast milk that have a deficiency in Vitamin D, may also develop this deficiency. This is very serious and potentially devastating for the developing fetus.

Another serious concern is that some pregnancies are unplanned and this means if the mother isn't getting enough sunshine, dietary Vitamin D or supplementation, she could be harming her fetus unknowingly.

Let's look into the problems at hand if a pregnant woman is lacking in Vitamin D:

* Gestational diabetes
* MS - multiple sclerosis
* Infertility - such as failed implantation
* Pre-eclampsia - dangerously high blood pressure during pregnancy
* Forced caesarean section delivery - increased by up to four hundred percent
* Vaginal infections - yeast
* Immunity issues

These are serious, but preventable issues for the most part. This makes it even more important that pregnant women take care of themselves. Not just when they are pregnant but well before the time they expect to get pregnant.

Experts are recommending that pregnant and lactation women get more than recommended in general for their Vitamin D intake. It's not unheard of to take between 6 and 8 000 IU/day.

Studies have also been shown that verify these higher doses of Vitamin D are not cause for concern. Because Vitamin D can be naturally manufactured by your body through sunshine, you've got built in safety mechanisms to ensure you don't get overdosed.

What's interesting to note is that British studies have found that children born to mothers that had low levels of Vitamin D throughout pregnancy, were more likely to be chubby. Moving on, we find out that babies from moms that had adequate amounts of Vitamin D were leaner.

Also, when the children reached age six, the ones that came from moms lacking Vitamin D, they seemed to have excess body fat. In other words, children seem to be pre-disposed to gain more fat if they don't get the Vitamin D they need in utero.

On another note, the Canadian Paediatric Society is pushing towards pregnant and lactating women to get up to ten times the daily recommended amount. And this might not even be enough to protect against chronic diseases.
It's also important to note that obese mothers may have even more of a difficult time ensuring their little ones get enough Vitamin D.

Lacking in Vitamin D isn't just linked to health issues. Experts have also found that children with language issues are more likely to have mothers that didn't get the Vitamin D they needed during pregnancy for various reasons.

Here researchers found that low Vitamin D in pregnancy likely means more problems in for the future for children. It is imperative that expecting mothers get the Vitamin D they need, so their baby has the best start possible!

My Thoughts . . .

Pregnant moms have a lot more to think about than just themselves. They need to make sure they do everything in their power to offer the best start for their baby.
Have a blood test performed to ensure you've got adequate amounts of Vitamin D in your blood, so that your growing baby is getting everything it needs. And upping your intake while pregnant is a good choice, just to ensure you are shorting yourself of your baby.

Final Thoughts . . .

You are in charge of you and taking the time to make certain you are getting all the Vitamin D you need is your responsibility. Keep yourself informed and up to date on what new research is arising and what experts are saying.

Your health is ever-changing and this means the amounts and methods of getting vitamins and minerals into your body are always going to be changing too.

You absorb Vitamin D differently than an infant does, or your friendly neighbor for that matter. Maybe you feel better with a specific type of supplement or make it a priority to get your Vitamin D each day with a little bit of sunshine, and live in the climate that accommodate this easily.

If you are predisposed to serious health issues, it may take a little more tinkering to get the Vitamin D into your system that you need. You may be wise to experiment a little to find whether sunshine, diet, supplementation, or a combination works best for you.

A simple blood test will give you all the information you need to be certain.

Life is what you make it and letting a little sunshine in is going to increase the odds that you are going to live a long and happy, happy, happy life. Sound good to you?